## DISCLAIMER

The information in this book is not intended as medical advice. The content is for information and research purposes only.

By reading this disclaimer, you fully accept the terms of this disclaimer. If you are not in agreement with this disclaimer, please do not order or read this book. The content of this book is provided for information and educational purposes only. Kindly do not interpret this book or its content for a medication or product. This is only a book guide.

Thanks

# Table of Contents

# INTRODUCTION

Whatever happens in our lives impacts our mind either consciously or unconsciously. Sometimes events such as the unexpected death of a loved one, illness, fearful thoughts, near-death accidents or experiences result in traumas. Psychological trauma causes damage to the psyche that occurs as a result of a severely distressing event.

Somatic psychotherapy is one of the best ways to help patients suffering from psychological traumas cope, recover and live a normal life. The word somatic is derived from the Greek word "soma" which means living body. Somatic therapy is a holistic therapy that studies the relationship between the mind and body in regard to psychological past. The theory behind somatic therapy is that trauma symptoms are the effects of instability of the ANS (autonomic nervous system). Past traumas disrupt the ANS.

According to somatic psychologists, our bodies hold on to past traumas which are reflected in our body language, posture and also expressions. In some cases past traumas may manifest physical symptoms like pain, digestive issues, hormonal imbalances, sexual dysfunction and immune system dysfunction, medical issues, depression, anxiety and addiction.

However, through somatic psychotherapy the ANS can again return to homeostasis. This therapy has been found to be quite useful in providing relief to disturbed patients and treating many physical and mental symptoms resulting from past traumas.

Somatic psychology confirms that the mind and body connection is deeply rooted. In recent years neuroscience has emerged with evidence that supports somatic psychology, showing how the mind influences the body and how the body influences the mind.

## Somatic Symptoms Disorder

Somatic symptom disorder (SSD formerly known as "somatization disorder" or "somatoform disorder") is a form of mental illness that causes one or more bodily symptoms, including pain. The symptoms may or may not be traceable to a physical cause including general medical conditions, other mental illnesses, or substance abuse. But regardless, they cause excessive and disproportionate levels of distress.

You often think the worst about your symptoms and frequently seek medical care, continuing to search for an explanation even when other serious conditions have been excluded. Health concerns may become such a central focus of your life that it's hard to function, sometimes leading to disability.

If you have somatic symptom disorder, you may experience significant emotional and physical distress. Treatment can help ease symptoms, help you cope and improve your quality of life.

## Symptoms

Symptoms of somatic symptom disorder may be:

- Specific sensations, such as pain or shortness of breath, or more general symptoms, such as fatigue or weakness
- Unrelated to any medical cause that can be identified, or related to a medical condition such as cancer or heart disease, but more significant than what's usually expected
- A single symptom, multiple symptoms or varying symptoms
- Mild, moderate or severe

Pain is the most common symptom, but whatever your symptoms, you have excessive thoughts, feelings or behaviors related to those symptoms, which cause significant problems, make it difficult to function and sometimes can be disabling.

These thoughts, feelings and behaviors can include:

- Constant worry about potential illness
- Viewing normal physical sensations as a sign of severe physical illness
- Fearing that symptoms are serious, even when there is no evidence
- Thinking that physical sensations are threatening or harmful
- Feeling that medical evaluation and treatment have not been adequate
- Fearing that physical activity may cause damage to your body
- Repeatedly checking your body for abnormalities
- Frequent health care visits that don't relieve your concerns or that make them worse

- Being unresponsive to medical treatment or unusually sensitive to medication side effects
- Having a more severe impairment than is usually expected from a medical condition

For somatic symptom disorder, more important than the specific physical symptoms you experience is the way you interpret and react to the symptoms and how they impact your daily life.

## Conditions Related to Somatic Symptom Disorder

### Anxiety

Anxiety disorders form a category of mental health diagnoses that lead to excessive nervousness, fear, apprehension, and worry

These disorders alter how a person processes emotions and behave, also causing physical symptoms. Mild anxiety might be vague and unsettling, while severe anxiety may seriously affect day-to-day living.

Somatic symptoms are the physical symptoms related to an illness. When the somatic symptoms of anxiety interfere with the activities of someone's life, that individual is considered to have an illness called generalized anxiety disorder.

**Kinds of Anxiety Disorder**

Generalized anxiety disorder: This is a chronic disorder involving excessive, long-lasting anxiety and worries about nonspecific life events, objects, and situations. GAD is the most common anxiety disorder, and people with the disorder are not always able to identify the cause of their anxiety.

**Panic disorder:** Brief or sudden attacks of intense terror and apprehension characterize panic disorder. These attacks can lead to shaking, confusion, dizziness, nausea, and breathing difficulties. Panic attacks tend to occur and escalate rapidly, peaking after 10 minutes. However, a panic attack might last for hours.

Panic disorders usually occur after frightening experiences or prolonged stress but may also occur without a trigger. An individual experiencing a panic attack may misinterpret it as a life-threatening illness, and may make drastic changes in behavior to avoid future attacks.

**Specific phobia:** This is an irrational fear and avoidance of a particular object or situation. Phobias are not like other anxiety disorders, as they relate to a specific cause.

A person with a phobia might acknowledge a fear as illogical or extreme but remain unable to control feelings anxiety around the trigger. Triggers for a phobia range from situations and animals to everyday objects.

**Agoraphobia:** This is a fear and avoidance of places, events, or situations from which it may be difficult to escape or in which help would not be available if a person becomes trapped. People often misunderstand this condition as a phobia of open spaces and the outdoors, but it is not so simple. A person with agoraphobia may have a fear of leaving home or using elevators and public transport.

**Selective mutism:** This is a form of anxiety that some children experience, in which they are not able to speak in certain places or contexts, such as school, even though they may have excellent verbal communication skills around familiar people. It may be an extreme form of social phobia.

**Social anxiety disorder, or social phobia:** This is a fear of negative judgment from others in social situations or of public embarrassment. Social anxiety disorder includes a range of feelings, such as stage fright, a fear of intimacy, and anxiety around humiliation and rejection.

This disorder can cause people to avoid public situations and human contact to the point that everyday living is rendered extremely difficult.

**Separation anxiety disorder:** High levels of anxiety after separation from a person or place that provides feelings of security or safety characterize separation anxiety disorder. Separation might sometimes result in panic symptoms.

Illness anxiety disorder is similar to somatic symptom disorder in that it requires a person to have a high level of anxiety about physical symptoms and to take disproportionate action in response to them. However, it is different from somatic symptom disorder in that it has more to do with how a person perceives an illness than with their actual symptoms. It is also more explicitly psychological in nature.

To be diagnosed with illness anxiety disorder, a person must exhibit the following symptoms:

- Preoccupation with having or developing a serious illness
- A lack of somatic symptoms or only mild symptoms and a disproportionate fear of their significance
- High levels of anxiety about health and alarmed reactions to perceived physical changes
- Excessive checking for symptoms or avoidance of any medical examination whatsoever
- Persistent preoccupation with these concerns that lasts at least six months

Illness anxiety disorder has two subtypes: care-seeking and care-avoiding. These subtypes are assigned based on whether a person makes excessive efforts to be seen frequently by medical professionals or avoids them altogether.

**Highlights**

- Tightening in the chest,
- Sweating,
- Jumping or feeling startled from noises or sounds,
- Diarrhea,
- Rapid heart rate,
- Shortness of breath,
- Problems concentrating,
- Problems falling asleep, and
- Very tense muscles.

**Depression**

Depression is a mood disorder that involves a persistent feeling of sadness and loss of interest. It is different from the mood fluctuations that people regularly experience as a part of life.

Major life events, such as bereavement or the loss of a job, can lead to depression. However, doctors only consider feelings of grief to be part of depression if they persist.

Depression is an ongoing problem, not a passing one. It consists of episodes during which the symptoms last for at least 2 weeks. Depression can last for several weeks, months, or years.

**Somatic Symptoms of Depression**

The term 'somatic symptom' is used loosely with respect to depression. Even researchers don't agree on exactly how to term these symptoms in general and exactly which specific symptoms should be included. Alternative terms that have been used in literature to refer to somatic symptoms or various groups of somatic symptoms include:

- Psychosomatic
- Somatoform

- Somatized
- Somatization
- Vegetative
- Masked

With respect to depression, somatic symptoms can be defined as bodily sensations that are either unpleasant or worrisome. These symptoms may affect one specific part of the body or they can affect the entire body.

Some potentially painful examples are headaches, backaches, general muscle pain and digestive pain like stomach pain.

Others might not be painful but are still unpleasant, like dizziness, dyspnea (or shortness of breath), and palpitations.

Some may affect the entire body, like fatigue or general weakness. Others involve changes in a person's appetite or even libido.

If you think that depression is solely or mainly a mental disorder with few to no somatic symptoms, you'd be wrong. In fact, almost 70% of people with depression go to the doctor because of their somatic symptoms, complaining of general aches and pain that are at least mildly severe.

**Factitious Disorder**

Factitious disorder is not a psychosomatic or medical condition but is a psychological condition in which a person claims to have physical or psychological symptoms they do not have. For a person to be diagnosed with the disorder, they must demonstrate all of the following:

- Falsification of physical or psychological symptoms
- Self-presentation as having an illness, impairment or injury
- Persistent deceptive behavior even in the absence of obvious external rewards

These symptoms cannot be better explained by another psychological condition, such as a psychotic or delusional disorder. The initial reason for the deception can vary, but the false symptoms persist even in the absence of financial gain or other external rewards. This clinical judgment distinguishes this disorder from malingering, the term used by providers to indicate that someone is intentionally falsifying an illness for an external reward.

People with factitious disorders are often motivated by a wish that they had another disorder. They want to be seen as having a particular medical or mental health condition and frequently have a history of child abuse or trauma. They may have genuine pain they want to heal but don't know how to express it directly. Sometimes people with factitious disorder induce symptoms of illness or injuries. They are often unaware that they are doing this.

## Conversion Disorder

Conversion disorder, also known as functional neurological symptom disorder, is the classic diagnosis for psychosomatic conditions. To be diagnosed with this condition, a person must:

- Have one or more symptoms of altered voluntary motor or sensory functions
- Have been examined by physicians who found that these physical symptoms were not compatible with any existing neurological or medical conditions
- Have symptoms that are not better explained by another medical or psychiatric condition

These symptoms must cause significant functional impairment or distress. Conversion disorder has several subtypes based on the nature of psychosomatic symptoms. Different categories of conversion disorder symptoms include the following:

- Weakness or paralysis
- Abnormal movement (such as tremor or altered gait)
- Swallowing symptoms
- Speech symptoms
- Attacks or seizures
- Anesthesia or sensory loss
- Special sensory symptoms (such as visual or hearing disturbance)
- Mixed symptoms

Psychological stressors can precipitate the condition or these symptoms can arise independently of any stressors.

## Causes of Somatic Symptom Disorder

Causes of somatic symptom and related disorders are as varied as the conditions themselves. Somatic symptom examples include exaggerated psychological reactions to medical conditions, psychosomatic symptoms and self-induced injury.

The causes of these symptoms and disorders are different but share certain factors in common.

**Genetic Causes**

Somatic symptom disorder symptoms may be particularly linked to family influence. Genetic factors affect how people perceive physical sensations, and family environments shape how people respond to these perceptions. A person is much more likely to develop a somatic disorder if they grew up with family members who had serious medical conditions or symptoms.

Similarly, the factitious disorder has been linked with having family members who are frequently hospitalized or are chronically ill. People learn from family members how much to fear illness and if medical symptoms are rewarded with special attention and care. Families who are unduly demonstrative of illness may inadvertently encourage members to view being ill as desirable.

## Biological Causes

Somatic symptom disorder with predominant pain is an example of a somatic condition driven by biological causes. Differences in brain chemistry and nervous system sensitivity can cause some people to have a heightened perception of pain. People with a heightened awareness of physical sensations may be more likely to interpret them as signs of a medical illness.

Research shows that BH4, a chemical produced by the nervous system, causes people to experience pain more intensely. People whose bodies produce more of this chemical have heightened reactions to pain because they experience it more acutely than others. Such sensitivities may especially influence the development of somatic symptom disorder and illness anxiety disorder.

## Psychological Causes (Hypochondriasis)

Somatic symptom disorder signs and symptoms can also come from purely psychological causes. Psychosomatic symptoms can develop in response to trauma or abuse. Some people convert psychological pain into physical symptoms through an unconscious process that helped them survive in a home in which emotional expression was discouraged or repressed. Factitious and conversion disorders can follow from frequent childhood experiences of being unable to receive psychological comfort or help.

Co-occurring psychiatric conditions can also contribute to the development of somatic symptom disorders. The anxiety that particular symptoms are worse than they are or fears they are harbingers of doom may be driven by comorbid anxiety disorders. Factitious and conversion disorders are sometimes linked to comorbid dissociative or personality disorders. Many trauma-related disorders, especially dissociative disorders, involve altered perceptions of bodily sensations and diminished or heightened reactions to them.

## How is Somatic Symptom Disorder Diagnosed?

Like most other psychiatric conditions, somatic symptom disorders are diagnosed through clinical interviews that confirm whether a person meets the relevant diagnostic criteria. Unlike other psychiatric conditions, these disorders often involve careful screening tests to determine whether physical symptoms have a medical origin.

Somatic symptom disorder tests are clinical instruments that may be used to determine whether reported physical symptoms arise from a medical condition or somatic disorder. Many clinicians use specific diagnostic instruments as part of an evaluation. These might include open-ended questions, multiple-choice questions or rating scales. The eight-item Somatic Symptom Scale (SSS-8) is a shortened form of the patient health questionnaire (PHQ) that was found to be a valid assessment tool in clinical research.

## Who is at Risk for Somatic Symptom Disorder?

Shared risk factors for somatic symptom disorder and related disorders include the following:

- A history of child abuse
- A history of traumatic experiences
- A history of childhood illness or of having a seriously ill parent
- Heightened sensitivity to physical sensations, especially pain
- Difficulty processing emotions or decreased awareness of them
- Comorbid anxiety, depression or dissociative disorders

- A prolonged period of heightened or acute stress

In general, people are at risk for somatic symptom disorders when they are more sensitive to physical sensations, grow up in families significantly affected by medical conditions and have histories of trauma or anxiety.

## Prevention

Little is known about how to prevent somatic symptom disorder. However, these recommendations may help.

- If you have problems with anxiety or depression, seek professional help as soon as possible.
- Learn to recognize when you're stressed and how this affects your body — and regularly practice stress management and relaxation techniques.

- If you think you have somatic symptom disorder, get treatment early to help stop symptoms from getting worse and impairing your quality of life.

- Stick with your treatment plan to help prevent relapses or worsening of symptoms.

## SOMATIC PSYCHOTHERAPY

Somatic psychotherapy, a holistic therapeutic approach, incorporates a person's mind, body, spirit, and emotions in the healing process. Proponents of this type of therapy believe a person's thoughts, attitudes, feelings, and beliefs can have an impact on physical functioning, while physical factors such as diet, exercise, and posture may positively or negatively affect a person's mental and emotional state. Thus, thoseseeking treatment for any number of mental health concerns may incorporating somatic therapy into treatment to be beneficial.

## What Is Somatic Psychotherapy?

A modality grounded in the mind-body connection, somatic psychotherapy is the largest branch of somatic psychology. Contemporary practitioners of somatic therapy believe that viewing the mind and body as one entity is essential to the therapeutic process. This mind/body entity will move toward healing and growth of its own accord, given the right environment, and interpersonal interactions, when conducted in a safe and respectful manner, can positively impact and help regulate the mind/body.

According to somatic therapy theory, the sensations associated with past trauma may become trapped within the body and reflected in facial expressions, posture, muscular pain, or other forms of body language. Talk therapy can help address this trauma, but depending on the needs of the person in treatment, therapeutic body techniques can supplement more conventional approaches (such as talking therapy) to provide holistic healing.

Somatic psychotherapy (also known as body psychotherapy or body-oriented psychotherapy) differs from body therapy. While body psychotherapy may often result in increased self-awareness, the resolution of psychological concerns, and positive changes in behavior, body therapy does not seek to resolve deep-rooted mental health issues or provide psychological insights. On the contrary, body therapy typically involves the use of therapeutic massage, non-therapeutic massages, and cosmetic skin treatments to reduce stress and increase long-term health.

**Essential Concepts of Body Psychotherapy.**

- **Bodymind:** Perhaps the most foundational concept of body psychotherapy, the bodymind represents the embodied integration of thoughts, feelings, and physical bodily experiences and sensations. All parts of a person can be accessed at various points in treatment in order to effectively and holistically address concerns. The „Bodymind" concept claims that our body is „living memory" and carries in it the signs and traces of our personal life experience as well as our familial heritage. All sorts of traumatic experiences and learned fears, impregnate our character and influence our posture which are tangible entrances to the whole Bodymind.

• **Armoring and Character:** Armoring is a concept developed by Reich. He believed people developed systems of bodily "armor," or muscle tension/rigidity, in order to protect themselves from emotional and physical pain. These sets of armor contribute to the development of a person's "character," according to Reich and his followers, who developed five basic character types to use during assessment and treatment.

• **Energy:** The concept of energy is central to the application of body psychotherapy. Energy metabolism, storage in and release from the body play an important role in how people carry themselves, hold themselves, experience and heal from pain, and interact with the world. Things like energy flow and release, pulsation, expansion and contraction (e.g. in tissues and organs), and energy charge and discharge are all things body psychotherapists pay attention to throughout treatment.

• **Body Memory:** This is the controversial premise that memories can actually be stored within the body. Body psychotherapists believe that because of this, some memories cannot be processed through talk therapy, but that these traumatic memories and problematic tension can often be released through bodywork and other physical techniques.

- **Trauma:** Body psychotherapy's concept of trauma aligns with that of body memory, proposing that traumatic experiences can create energy build-up, or blockages, that lead to physical and mental health concerns.

## How Somatic Psychotherapy Works

While traditional talk therapies are often able to effectively address many mental and emotional health challenges, somatic psychotherapists believe some people may be able to quickly address deep emotional issues not revealed through talk therapy, simply by paying attention to the communication of the body. Because past trauma or other psychological concerns may potentially have a negative effect on a person's autonomic nervous system, people experiencing emotional and psychological issues may also be affected by physical concerns such as sexual dysfunction, hormonal issues, digestive issues, or tension in specific parts of the body such as the head, neck, shoulders, or stomach.

Practitioners of somatic psychotherapy can help individuals both become more aware of these bodily sensations and learn to use therapeutic techniques to release any tension the body is holding. Techniques often used in therapy include breathing exercise and sensation awareness, physical exercise such as dance or other movement, voice work, massage, and grounding exercises. During the session, the person in treatment may be encouraged to reflect on patterns of behavior and identify any impact these patterns may have on any new emotions, experiences, or concerns that come up in therapy.

## How Can Somatic Psychotherapy Help?

Somatic therapy may help people experience greater self-awareness and connection to others. Participants may find themselves able to better sense their own bodies, reduce stress, and explore emotional and physical concerns.

The use of body-oriented psychotherapies as part of an integrated approach to the treatment of posttraumatic stress is becoming more prevalent and trauma experts has stated that somatic approaches may in fact be essential in trauma treatment.

Somatic psychotherapy can help individuals address a range of issues. Some may choose to seek somatic therapy as part of their approach to treatment in order to improve emotional regulation, address relationship concerns, decrease symptoms of anxiety or depression, and increase self-confidence. Scientific evidence supporting this treatment is limited, but early research suggests somatic therapies may also be helpful when included in the treatment of issues such as borderline personality.

## Patient Story

James is a 36-year-old married male who has been seen by Dr. Donald, a primary care physician who practices near James's work. James began to see Dr. Donald three months ago after abdominal pain he had been experiencing for about a year was becoming progressively worse. James noticed that the abdominal pain would come on intermittently, was located everywhere in his abdomen and was not consistently related to food intake. He tried changing his diet and cutting out dairy products, wheat products and even meat, but nothing seemed to help. He quit drinking any alcohol or caffeine, and the pain only seemed to become more frequent and severe. Before he went to see Dr. Donald, the pain had become so bad that he had missed a few days at work and had cancelled an outing with his wife and friends to a popular camping spot because he was afraid he would have another "attack".

Dr. Donald saw James and performed a thorough physical exam and a detailed history of the entire course of James's symptoms. Dr. Donald asked James about unrelated symptoms, and ordered some laboratory tests to evaluate for autoimmune disorders and check his overall health, which all came back very normal. Dr. Donald phoned James and asked him to keep a log of his symptoms and anything that was related to bringing them in, and after reviewing the log together at their next appointment, Dr. Donald and James could not identify any other clues as to what was happening.

Nevertheless, James seemed to be preoccupied with these symptoms, and Dr. Donald noted how debilitating they were to James. Dr. Donald was able to reflect on just how often James was fearful of the onset of the symptoms, and noted that James's wife felt like she'd lost her husband.

Dr. Donald scheduled a special meeting to review with James all the progress they'd made together over the previous three months. They reviewed more testing they had ordered, including an ultrasound and some other lab tests which found nothing unusual. Dr. Donald, James and his wife all agreed that whatever was happening, James had lost his ability to be happy or have pleasure in any activities, and seemed to be suffering with a severe depression. They could also agree that Dr. Donald would continue to work with James to seek out new data and look for any other causes of his pain, while James would begin to work on learning to live with his pain and cope with it until something else changed.

After another three months, James felt that his mood was better after receiving several sessions of counseling and cognitive behavioral therapy specifically related to his pain, and was able to note that the frequency and the severity of his pain symptoms were better when he was consistently taking an antidepressant medication, which was nice. Although the pain wasn't gone, it seemed more manageable and James found that he was going out more with friends and his wife, and his wife seemed much happier. James and Dr. Donald still met regularly to review his progress and ensure that no new symptoms or changes to the character of his symptoms were occurring, and James found that he was gradually able to get back into his life, and, in doing so, found that his pain was getting better and much more tolerable.

## Concerns & Limitations

Despite its reported effectiveness and increasing popularity in therapy, some concerns have been raised regarding the use of somatic psychotherapy as a treatment option. One issue is the use of touch, which is utilized as part of some somatic approaches. Touch in therapy is a major ethical concern. While some individuals assert that therapeutic techniques involving physical contact with the therapist result in pain reduction and the release of tension, some people such as those affected by sexual abuse may have significant issues with being physically touched.

Some experts have also questioned whether the use of touch could have the unintended effect of rendering therapy sessions frightening, arousing, or sexual. The possible presence of these types of intense emotions could contribute to the development of greater transference and countertransference issues within the therapeutic relationship. In order for this type of treatment to be effective, both the therapist and the person in treatment must consent to touch and possess the capacity to learn how to develop their own bodily awareness.

Because not all forms of body psychotherapy have satisfied the tests for scientific validity posited by accrediting institutions in some countries, certain body-centered approaches may not be recognized or accepted within those countries.

## Lifestyle & Home Remedies

While somatic symptom disorder benefits from professional treatment, you can take some lifestyle and self-care steps, including these:

• Work with your care providers. Work with your medical care provider and mental health professional to determine a regular schedule for visits to discuss your concerns and build a trusting relationship. Also discuss setting reasonable limits on tests, evaluations and specialist referrals. Avoid seeking advice from multiple doctors or emergency room visits that can make your care more difficult to coordinate and may subject you to duplicate testing.

• Practice stress management and relaxation techniques. Learning stress management and relaxation techniques, such as progressive muscle relaxation, may help improve symptoms.

• Get physically active. A graduated activity program may have a calming effect on your mood, improve your physical symptoms and help improve your physical function.

• Participate in activities. Stay involved in your work and in social and family activities. Don't wait until your symptoms are resolved to participate.

• Avoid alcohol and recreational drugs. Substance use can make your care more difficult. Talk to your health care provider if you need help quitting.

## Benefit of Somatic Exercises

The most important thing for you to remember is that Somatic Exercises change your muscular system by changing your central nervous system. If you do not remember this important fact, their effectiveness will be diminished for you.

You will receive the maximum benefit from the Somatic Exercise movement patterns if you do the following:

1. While doing the somatic exercises, your primary task is to focus your attention on the internal sensations of movement. These movement patterns highlight those areas of the body most commonly affected by sensory-motor amnesia. As you perform the exercises, concentrate on developing a careful

sensory awareness of the movements in these body areas as a direct way to maintain control over them.

2. Ideally, you should do your somatic exercises while lying on a rug or mat, wearing loose clothing and being away from all distractions. A rug or mat allows comfort while providing a firm support for your body. This allows you to be more precise in performing the movement and more precise in perceiving it. People whose movement or strength is extremely limited may do their Somatic Exercises in bed. The firmer their mattresses, the more effective the exercises will be, and they should move to a rug or mat as soon as possible.

The object of Somatic Exercises is to loosen your body from constricted muscles, so it makes no sense to wear constricting clothing while you do them. On the other hand, there's no need for athletic gear. You're not supposed to work up a sweat doing Somatic Exercises.

3. Always move slowly. Moving slowly, you give your brain the chance to notice all that is happening in your body as you move. Slow-motion films are essential in sports training because they allow athletes to study the details of a movement or play. The same goes for focusing attention on the internal sensations of your own movements: The slower you go, the more you perceive.

4. Always move gently and with the least possible effort. This again, is so that your brain can receive precise and uncluttered sensory feedback from the exercises. When you experience excessive effort and strain-as is usually the case in doing calisthenics-then your brain is cluttered by sensory feedback that is irrelevant to what you are relearning to control. It is better for you to feel that you are doing " too little" than to risk doing too much and undermining the somatic learning process.

5. Do not force any movement. Somatic Exercises help you maintain sensitivity and control, but, until your brain learns how to move your muscles, no amount of force and effort will release the involuntary contractions in your body. Pushing against your muscles is from the old tradition of physical training, which always fails to release the hold of sensory-motor amnesia. If you attempt to voluntarily force a muscle that is involuntarily contracted, you will cause an equal and opposite resistance of that muscle. It will contract even tighter, finally to the point of spasm.

Remember: If you want to untie a knot, you must look at the cord carefully then gently undo the tangle. Yanking on the cord will only make the knot tighter.

6. Somatic exercises are not painful.

The movement patterns of these exercises are the normal movements of the musculoskeletal system.

If you perform them slowly and gently, they are completely harmless. Hurting yourself while exercising is unnecessary harmful and, of course, no fun at all.

People who are already suffering from sensory-motor amnesia, especially those with severely contracted lower back muscles, will sometimes feel soreness when these muscles first begin to lengthen. This is to be expected; and once their muscles lengthen, the soreness will disappear. Even very painful lower back muscles become comfortable after about three days of Somatic Exercises, once they have relaxed to their natural length and blood has circulated through the muscle fibers. Thus, if you feel some pain doing the exercises, move gently and slowly, never forcing your movements, and keep in mind that this is the normal direction of movement that you are trying to reestablish.

There are always unusual situations where normal musculoskeletal movement patterns are impossible because of an observable obstacle. In such cases, you should seek medical advice and follow it. Physicians usually agree that Somatic Exercises are anatomically harmless when done properly.

7. Be persistent, patient, and positive somatic exercises change your body by teaching your brain. Your learning grows steadily and solidly. You must be persistent determined in your practice of these movement patterns. You must be patient looking not for a quick fix on your body, but for a genuine, lasting change in your comfort, range of movement, posture, and general functioning. Most importantly, you must be positive in your expectations, envisaging and aiming for the improvement you know your somatic system is capable of.

8. Learn the nature of sensory-motor amnesia, how it occurs in your brain, and where it occurs in your body.

## A 6-step Somatic Healing

### 1. Notice.

Inhale and exhale, notice what you feel on, in and around your body. Speed of breath, heart rate and body temperature.

### 2. Think back to safety.

Think back to at a recent moment you felt most calm, safe and most like your "self".

### 3. Identify.

Identify at what point in time and/or which part of your body began experiencing disturbance or stress.

## 4. Replay.

Replay the scenario from calm state to stressed state, in slow motion (as if watching a slow movie). Identify people, conversations, objects or behaviors that may have made you stressed, uncomfortable or that stand out to you as you're replaying the recent event(s).

## 5. Tune in.

Tune in to your body sensations as you recall the event(s) and slow down and notice if there is any shift in your body, a sensation of tingling, tensing, warming, numbing or cooling in your chest, arms, legs, face or an overall change in body temperature.

## 6. Healing hands.

Place your hand on the area that has experienced a shift or change, and breathe deeply. If it's an overall feeling, you can simply place your hands on your heart.

Doing this allows the body to process the somatic experience, and creates a passageway to release the tension.

Notice if something comes up, an image, sensation, awareness or understanding that offers clarity to the situation. If nothing comes up, that's ok. Simply slowing down, pacing your breath and raising awareness is progress and helpful in itself.

I encourage you to practice this after an upsetting experience, to allow your body to process the emotions and communications of your body. You may also choose to practice this before a stressful situation so that you can identify potential triggers and plan ahead ways to support yourself.

As you go about your day, I encourage you to tune in to your body.

It is important to note that this exercise is not in place of trauma therapy; rather it is a skill you can practice on your own adjunctive to good therapy work. If you are in therapy and notice something new while doing this exercise, jot it down and bring it to your therapist for deeper and continued work. if you are not in therapy and realize that a lot has come up for you, I encourage you to begin your healing today.

Counseling can help you release the tension and somatic stress carried on your body.

If you have been experiencing tension, anxiety, or trauma symptoms that express themselves in the body, due to something from the past, or specific to something that's come up, I encourage you to reach out to a therapist today.

## CBD Oil Indication in Treating Somatic Symptoms Disorder

There is also evidence drawn from preclinical trials of CBD that the substance could be useful in treating anxiety disorders, which makes it a conceivably attractive option in psychosomatic disorder treatment as well., CBD could potentially assist with both somatic and psychological issues at once, treating both anxiety and the physical pain simultaneously. In regards to strictly somatic pain, CBD shows potential as well. Though research is lacking, some users claim that CBD in topical lotions, applied locally, may assist with minor aches and pains. Ultimately, more research must be concluded before the efficacy of CBD as a psychological-, psychosomatic-, and somatic-pain management solution is established. Nevertheless, CBD-derived oils and lotions have been gaining popularity in the U.S. in this regard, and, as regulations surrounding cannabis and derivative products have loosened, public and private interests in these products has grown and likely will continue to.

# CONCLUSION



Somatic therapy can be integrated into other psychotherapy and counseling practices. Look for a licensed, experienced mental health professional with advanced, supervised training in somatic therapy techniques. In addition to finding someone with the appropriate educational background, experience and positive approach, look for a therapist with whom you feel comfortable discussing personal issues.